NATURAL POTENCY - WHAT TO DO IF YOUR »BEST PART« IS ON STRIKE?

NATURAL POTENCY-ENHANCING REMEDIES TO INCREASE VIRILITY FROM THE ABILITY TO GET AN ERECTION TO STEADFASTNESS

DIETER MANN

ISBN 978-1-63886-836-1

Contents

Preface

Dear reader,

To many of us, virility is more than just a physical function, such as digestion or the ability to distinguish different flavors from each other. To many men, virility represents the core of their »manhood«. Where it is limited or where it even disappeared completely, many men feel deprived of their masculinity.

While it is perfectly normal for women that they at a certain point in life lose the ability to bear children, men think about the loss of the ability to reproduce as the beginning of their end. It is obvious that this is not about the wish of the majority of men to father a child at the age of sixty, seventy or eighty. It is rather the sole ability (potency), to do it, which represents an important feature of manhood in our society.

It is exactly this circumstance from which some producers of treatment for impotence (think for example of the well-known blue pills), but also producers of ineffective »miracle cures« made from tiger penises or rhinoceros horns, benefit.

While former show a lot of side effects, the latter has no effect at all. Both, however, cost a lot - and it almost seems as if we thought that what costs a lot also has a big effect.

In fact, natural potency-enhancing drugs, that for one have almost or completely no side effects and at the same time are high quality and cost only a fraction of the formerly mentioned products, have been known for centuries. This book is dedicated to exactly these little-known »magic cures« from nature and, of course, to you as the reader. Regardless of whether you want to take precautions or need to resolve an existing problem. In this book, you will find interesting information.

Have great joy with your manhood!

Dieter Mann

All information that is presented in this books has been researched in all conscience. But they do not replace professional advice from skilled experts in any way and do not promise a cure for your problem. It is strongly advised to everyone to consult a physician of your choice before taking any type of medication, regardless of whether it is of chemical or natural origin.

CHAPTER ONE

SOLUTIONS FROM THE TEST TUBE

Just like handkerchiefs are often designated with the trade name Tempo, it is the same for chemical treatment of impotence and the product name »Viagra®«. Only a few people are aware of the fact that by now there exist quite a few other, similarly positioned pharmaceutical drugs on the market. Cialis® and Levitra® are the most famous among them.

Regarding the history of Viagra Wikipedia says:

In the early 1990s, a team of researchers of a Pfizer research institute in Sandwich sought for a remedy for curing heart trouble. The remedy UK-92480, which was found within this context, blocked the enzyme PDE-5. While initial tests on patients were very promising, some men reported multiple erections a few days after the intake of the medication. The concerned examiner saw no potential in the effect; therefore, Pfilzer filed a patent application for the active agent as sildenafil citrate in 1991.

After the medication for heart trouble turned out to have no effect, the sexual effect of the active agent was considered more in detail. In a study conducted on 300 men in England, France, and Sweden 90 percent reported having erections; hardly any side effects were observed. In 1998, Pfilzer got permission of the US health authority to sell Viagra. Time magazine reported about the potency pill in a cover story.

In 2003, two other medications with the same mechanism of action were launched. Levita (Bayer) and Cialis (Eli Lilly). In 2012 another active agent with the name Avanafil (Mitsubishi Pharma), which is supposed to show an effect faster than Viagra, followed. The trade name is Stendra. Since April 2014 Spendra (Berlin-Chemie with the active agent avanafil) is available in Germany.

In 2007, Pfizer captured a market share of 47 percent on the world market for substances against erectile dysfunction, in 2013 it had 36 percent. In 2012, Pfizer generated a revenue of two billion US-dollars.

Obviously, this is about a huge amount. With this, we speak about an economic performance of some countries of the Third World, which corresponds to the revenue of the world market leader of the blue pills alone. Of course, it is up to the user himself, if he is willing to pay the demanded price for the temporary optimization of his ability to get an erection.

Many men, who are partly not willing to pay the demanded price at a pharmacy or who feel embarrassed, get the mentioned products, especially the »blue pills«, from the internet or from street vendors or local suppliers from dubious markets on journeys abroad. One can only hope that they fell for colored and pressed corn sugar because all other alternatives are potentially damaging to one's health or fatal.

The products which are available on the gray market are partly characterized by foreign admixtures and cutting agents or by incorrect dosages. Sometimes even completely different substances, which are just pressed into the familiar form, are offered. Literally everything can be contained.

Even if one assumes that the buyer actually purchased the real substance - the chances for that are within a range of one-figure thousands - he still faces a not to be underestimated danger. The number of contraindications - that means those cases of application in which the products are damaging to one's health or even fatal -is remarkable. There are even phraseologies in the package inserts of some products such as »if you have or once had low blood pressure«.

That means that the producer concerned makes clear that men who at some point in their life had low blood pressure could suffer damage by ingesting the product.

Fact is that there is hardly anyone who has never had low blood pressure as a result of an illness or due to other circumstances. Only a physician who knows all health-related facts can correctly assess this and the many other medical reasons, which militate against a usage of respective products. Cases in which the miracle pill was used on one's own responsibility despite the contraindications can be found in newspaper reports again and again. Newspapers then report about people who died during or after sexual intercourse or who experienced extensive health disorders.

Eventually und finally, it can be said that taking the expensive miracle pills will not be successful for many men (studies say about 20-30%) and can lead to permanent erections for some others. This refers to a disorder that in most cases can only by corrected by surgery.

In no way an approved drug is supposed to be talked down with that. It only seems important that the consumer informs himself about the functioning, effect and side-effects of the medication before taking it and consults a physician for advice on any medical measures.

CHAPTER TWO

NATURAL REMEDIES

Natural remedies for sexual disorders have always existed, regardless of whether it was only about consuming substances or shamanic rituals. Men who did not »function« the way they wanted to have always looked for alternatives.

The following natural substances undoubtedly only represent an extract of available applications but give a good overview of what is possible.

It is strongly discouraged to take and purchase any miracle cures. Those who believe that taking tiger penis powder gives them the strength of a tiger or that consuming ground rhinoceros horn increases their steadfastness, must actually also believe that with eating a piece of beef they will start to moo and give milk.

Arginine

One of the most frequently offered natural remedy for men with potency problems is called L-arginine or short arginine. It is a substance that the human body can produce by itself. However, this is (often) not done in sufficient quantity, which is why the additional intake of arginine is also common in traditional medicine.

Arginine can be found in various foods that are consumed daily. A compilation of respective foods can be found on Wikipedia:

Food	Total protein	Arginine	Amount
Buckwheat grains	13,25 g	982 mg	7,4 %
Peas, dried	24,55 g	2188 mg	8,9 %
Peanuts, roasted	23,68 g	2832 mg	11,9 %
Chicken breast fillet, raw	21,23 g	1436 mg	6,8 %
Chicken egg	12,57 g	820 mg	6,5 %
Cow milk, 3,7 % Fat	3,28 g	119 mg	3,6 %
Pumpkin seeds	30,23 g	5353 mg	17,7 %
Salmon, raw	20,42 g	1221 mg	6,0 %

Food	Total protein	Arginine	Amount
Corn-wholemeal flour	6,93 g	345 mg	5,0 %
Pinekernels	13,69 g	2413 mg	17,6 %
Rice, unpeeled	7,94 g	602 mg	7,6 %
Pork, raw	20,95 g	1394 mg	6,7 %
Walnuts	15,23 g	2278 mg	15,0 %
Wheat-wholemeal flour	13,70 g	642 mg	4,7 %

Concerning erectile function, its mode of action is the following: To obtain a satisfactory erection, it is necessary for the blood vessels in the penis to get so wide that the cavernous body can be filled with enough blood. Nitric oxide (NO) is significantly involved in the dilatation of the vessels. However, it does not only improve the dilatation of the vessels but also perfusion and thus nutrient supply of the cells, which in turn has a positive effect on potency and the quality of the sperm.

Nitric oxide is produced from arginine within the body in only a few steps. The arginine can up to a certain extent be won from the above-mentioned foods with our body. In cases of increased strain, such as stress, the body can not cover the demand from only these sources. The amount of arginine that the body needs can also increase because of diseases such as high blood pressure, arteriosclerosis or erectile dysfunction.

Lately, arginine has been experiencing a real boom. This is because of positive studies and the almost complete absence of side effects and especially because it is a substance that a healthy body produces on its own and not an exogenous substance.

Many experts recommend using an activator when taking arginine, in order to accelerate the absorption of the substance. OPS and green tea extract haven proven to be particularly useful as activators.

When taking arginine, it is, of course, important to resort to high-quality products of leading producers. When comparing various offers one should pay special attention to the contained active ingredient concentration. Experts advice 3000-5000mg of arginine per day. In acute cases and after consulting an expert also daily allowances of 10,000 mg are possible. The effect should be noticeable after only a few days. Also not every active agent can trigger side effects and potential incompatibilities. It is therefore, in any case, advisable to consult a professional before consuming the substance.

Yohimbine

Yohimbine is extracted from the leaves and the bark of the Yohimbe tree (pausinystalia yohimbe). It is an alkaloid. Europeans have learned how to use the bark of the yohimbe tree from indigenous people from Central and West Africa where using it is widespread since »time immemorial«. The importance and interest was so great that already in 1890 a process of preparation of yohimbine was patented. Since then the remedy has been used to overcome impotence.

Even today, respective preparations are offered by several companies.

Yohimbine contains an alpha-2-receptor antagonist which has an effect on the brain as well as the vessels within the penis. In the brain, it has an effect on the erection-inhibiting, sympathetic nervous system which is for example active when one has fears of failure.

At the same time, it penetrates the blood-cerebral-barrier and leads to an increase in blood pressure and heart rate. The genital centers are aroused and an increase in the amount of blood that is pumped into the genital organs is triggered.

Yohimibine especially has an effect on psychologically caused potency problems, which for example are based on fears of failure. Yohimbine can be taken, depending on the intended goal, one to two hours before the intended intercourse or as part of a longer-term therapy over the course of two to eight weeks. Indication of quantity by the producer should not be exceeded.

Yohimbine, just like any substance that has an effect on the circulatory system, has various side effects and contraindications which should be discussed with a physician.

Maca

The maca plant which has its origin in Peru belongs to the group of the cress plants. In its habitat, it grows on plateaus at altitudes of about 4000 meters. The plant is optimally adapted to harsh weather conditions and poor soil. That is because the plant can store and enrich nutrients within its thickened root. Besides starch and sugar, it contains various essential amino acids and fats. In addition, it is rich in vitamins, mineral nutrients, trace elements and secondary plant compounds. In its place of origin, it is appreciated as a substantial food. Regarding the effect of the plant Wikipedia writes:

Positive effects on physical performance and psychological resilience are attributed to the maca root. According to clinical studies, this effect is not the result of an endocrinologic, that is hormonopoietic-processes-influencing, effect; a change in hormone levels in humans could not be observed. However, the plant seems to have a positive effect on sexual dysfunctions. Dietary supplements that contain maca powder have been on the market as natural impotence treatment in Europe and the US for some time past. As with many other products of this kind, these effects have not been entirely scientifically proven.

The supply via commercially available dietary supplements is well below the nutritional intake of the inhabitants of the Andes. Almost only the dried powder of the tuber is used.

Studies from South America and the United States (which are, however, more based on experience reports than on measurable data) show however that the probands reported an increase in sexual desire and performance, a stronger immune system, and more energy, moreover, it is supposed to counteract depression and chronic fatigue.

The Peruvian scientist Gustavo Gonzales gave maca to twelve men between 20 and 40 for three months and examined their fertility afterwards. Already after two weeks, he could on average determine a doubling in the amount of sperm. At the same time, male hormones were formed and the probands swore that their sexual desire had significantly increased.

Chinese scientists published a study where maca extract was given to mice, that were then able to have 47-67 orgasms within three hours. The mice of the control group only had 16 orgasms in the same time.

The neurologist Fernando Cabiesee, who also examined the potency-improving effect of maca, assessed that the plant does not only increase the ability to get an erection, but also the general drive to be sexually active over the long term.

Maca is offered in the market as the »natural Viagra«. In fact, it must rather be seen as a very original food which was grown and enjoyed by the natives of Peru during centuries and which has hoped-for side effects.

Various scientific studies show that taking maca over a longer period of time has an extremely positive effect. The result is an overproduction of hormones, for example also of testosterone. This hormone causes a boost of energy which can have a positive effect on the process of coping with negative external influences which trigger stress, depressions and anxiety.

It can be said that the effect of maca and Viagra® and similar products is entirely different. While the pills have a vasodilating effect, which has a direct impact on the penis and which leads to sexual stimulus right after taking them, maca addresses an increase in sexual drive and sustainable improvement of perfusion. One could compare both ways in a way that says that the chemical preparations rather offer assist-starting while maca starts with repairing the battery.

Maca root is used in natural medicine in the areas of increase in libido (sexual drive), improvement of steadfastness, ability to obtain an erection, improvement of quantity and quality of sperm, but also in the area of increasing the fertility of women and in order to prevent miscarriages.

Maca is offered on the market in the form of various preparations as powders, capsules and pressed. Because the consumed amount with this preparation is only a fraction of what is consumed in the country of its origin, it is not necessary to expect significant side effects. Nevertheless, it is recommended to observe the quality and to consult a physician for clarification of interactions with other products consumed and possible incompatibilities.

Ginseng

Ginseng is considered to be the Asian medical plant per se in the West. For over 2000 years it has been used in medicine. In consideration of its occurrence mainly in the mountain and forest regions of North Korea, north-eastern China, and south-eastern Siberia, the plant was for a long time reserved for the rich. However, the plant does only hardly ever occur in the wilderness anymore, so that the demand on the world market is rather covered by cultivated Ginseng. Its cultivation has been operated for more than 800 years and is very complex and expensive, especially as the roots of ginseng need five to six years in order to reach their potency of active ingredients.

On the market, white ginseng is distinguished from red ginseng even if they derive from the same plant and differ only in their processing. While white ginseng is peeled, bleached and dried right after harvesting it, the red ginseng firstly needs to be treated with steam.

The content of ginsenosides is crucial for the medical effect. It is influenced by age, cultivation region, soil quality and processing.

Primarily, ginseng is a roborant with a strong adaptogenic effect. In addition, it is also used as a natural and effective impotence treatment. Studies have shown that it has an effect on approximately two-thirds of all men.

As with maca the potency-enhancing effect is based mainly on the production of testosterone as well as the release of nitric oxide (NO), just as with arginine. Additionally, perfusion in the genital area is stimulated.

Ginseng has a very gentle positive effect on stress-related erectile dysfunction. Important with that is a sufficient dosage. A daily intake of 10mg ginsenosides is described as useful in specialized literature (roughly corresponds to 1-2g of high-quality ginseng root).

Ginkgo

Ginkgo is a type of tree from China that is nowadays grown worldwide. Mixed forest, but sometimes also mountain valleys were the original habitat.

Ginkgo is also called »living fossil« because it is the only survivor of its botanical group. It is a deciduous tree which can become older than thousand years and higher than 40 meters. Since the seeds can have an unpleasant odor of butyric acid, in Europe the tree is mainly spread as a male tree in the form of cuttings.

Only the leaves are used pharmaceutically. They have been used for over thousand years specifically in the form of special extracts. When processing them correctly, undesired side active agents are separated by extraction.

Ginkgo preparations have a neuroprotective effect; cognitive performance and learning ability are enhanced and flowing properties of the blood are optimized. For this reason, ginkgo is also used for preventing and treating dementia, for treating organically caused memory and concentration problems as well as for treating tinnitus, dizziness, and headache.

Ginkgo stimulates the blood flow, which has an extreme effect of relaxation of the muscles of the cavernous body within the penis. A longer-lasting and stronger erection is the result. Specialized literature constitutes amounts of 40-100mg of ginkgo extract as sufficient, whereas under medical supervision even amounts up to 240mg are possible.

Gingko has some known, rather rare side effects. In rare cases, gastrointestinal complaints and headaches have been observed. But it does exist a clear contraindication when taking blood-thinning medications.

CHAPTER THREE

ATTENTION DANGEROUS!

Unfortunately, new miracle cures, where the mode of action has not been proven and that only exist to take money from desperate men, are frequently offered on the market. Some do not even have an effect (or a completely different effect than desired), but some actually increase erection and desire, but after single intake already leads to lasting physical damages.

Equally dangerous are black market products, products from dubious senders and products from no-name producers. At best, you buy sugar pastilles for serious money - at worst, it is rat poison or any similar fatal product. Thus: Hands off!

Also always to note is the fact that overdoses or interactions with other preparations can lead to undesired consequences or even to serious damages to one's health. In any case, it is important to be moderate and to consult an expert before taking any preparation.

CHAPTER FOUR

VIRILITY AND PSYCHE

Just like many things in life, problems often begin with health-related challenges in one's head. Therefore, it is not surprising that experts maintain that in the majority of cases potency problems, reduced sex drive, lack of stamina or premature ejaculation have a more psychological than physical reason.

This is not surprising if one is aware of the fact that challenges, such as stress, anxiety, sleep deficit, overextension, erratic lifestyle and many others, of course, have an influence on our psyche and thus also indirectly on our body.

For this reason, also mental and psychological aspects should be taken into account in the context of a clean clarification of occurring problems.

And finally: A »real man« has undoubtedly more to offer to the world (and his partner) than some centimetres of flesh and skin. Do not worry »when it does not work for once«.

Have fun and good luck

Yours, Dieter Mann

Disclaimer

Introduction

By using this book, you accept this disclaimer in full.

No advice

The book contains information. The information is not advice and should not be treated as such.

No representations or warranties

To the maximum extent permitted by applicable law and subject to section below, we exclude all representations, warranties, undertakings and guarantees relating to the book.

Without prejudice to the generality of the foregoing paragraph, we do not represent, warrant, undertake or guarantee:

- that the information in the book is correct, accurate, complete or non-misleading.

- that the use of the guidance in the book will lead to any particular outcome or result.

Limitations and exclusions of liability

The limitations and exclusions of liability set out in this section and elsewhere in this disclaimer: are subject to section 6 below; and govern all liabilities arising under the disclaimer or in relation to the book, including liabilities arising in contract, in tort (including negligence) and for breach of statutory duty.

We will not be liable to you in respect of any losses arising out of any event or events beyond our reasonable control.

We will not be liable to you in respect of any business losses, including without limitation loss of or damage to profits, income, revenue, use, production, anticipated savings, business, contracts, commercial opportunities or goodwill.

We will not be liable to you in respect of any loss or corruption of any data, database or software.

We will not be liable to you in respect of any special, indirect or consequential loss or damage.

Exceptions

Nothing in this disclaimer shall: limit or exclude our liability for death or personal injury resulting from negligence; limit or exclude our liability for fraud or fraudulent misrepresentation; limit any of our liabilities in any way that is not permitted under applicable law; or exclude any of our liabilities that may not be excluded under applicable law.

Severability

If a section of this disclaimer is determined by any court or other competent authority to be unlawful and/or unenforceable, the other sections of this disclaimer continue in effect.

If any unlawful and/or unenforceable section would be lawful or enforceable if part of it were deleted, that part will be deemed to be deleted, and the rest of the section will continue in effect.

Law and jurisdiction

This disclaimer will be governed by and construed in accordance with Swiss law, and any disputes relating to this disclaimer will be subject to the exclusive jurisdiction of the courts of Switzerland.

9 781638 868361